DK Natural Care Library

SAW PALMETTO

HORMONE HEALTH ENHANCER

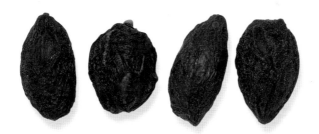

By STEPHANIE PEDERSEN

DORLING KINDERSLEY PUBLISHING, INC.

www.dk.com

CONTENTS

HERBAL HISTORY

Long before over-the-counter medications and prescription drugs came on the scene, herbs proved to be powerful healers. Every culture on earth has used herbal medicine. In fact, herbal usage is older than recorded history itself: Herbal preparations were found in the burial site of a Neanderthal man who lived over 60,000 years ago.

When it comes to herbal medicine, many healing systems are available and useful. Perhaps the best known are ayurveda, Chinese medicine, and Western herbalism. Ayurveda is a system of diagnosis and treatment that uses herbs in conjunction with breathing, meditation, and yoga. It has been practiced in India for more than 2,500 years. Ayurveda gets its name from the Sanskrit words *ayuh*, meaning "longevity," and *veda*, meaning "knowledge." Indeed, in ayurvedic healing, health can be achieved only after identifying a person's physical and mental characteristics (called *dosha*). Then the proper preventative or therapeutic remedies are prescribed to help an individual maintain doshic balance.

Chinese medicine is another healing system that uses herbs, in combination with acupressure, acupuncture, and qi gong. Sometimes called traditional Chinese medicine (TCM), this ancient system is thought to be rooted as far back as 2,800 BC in the time of emperor Sheng Nung. Known as China's patron saint of herbal medicine, Sheng Nung is credited among the first proponents of healing plants. Chinese medicine attempts to help the body correct energy imbalances. Therefore herbs are classified according to certain active characteristics, such as heating, cooling, moisturizing, or drying, and prescribed according to how they influence the activity of various organ systems.

Many herbal practitioners believe that Western herbalism can trace its roots to the ancient Sumerians, who—according to a medicinal recipe dating from 3000 BC—boasted a refined knowledge of herbal medicine. Records from subsequent cultures, such as the Assyrians, Egyptians, Israelites, Greeks, and Romans, show similar herbal healing systems. But these peoples weren't the only ones using beneficial plants. The Celts, Gauls, Scandinavians, and other early European tribes also healed with herbs. In fact, it was their knowledge, melded with the medicine brought by invading Moors and Romans, that formed the foundation for Western herbalism. Simply put, this foundation formed a comprehensive system wherein herbs were grouped according to how they affected both the body and specific body systems.

Western herbalism was refined further when Europeans traveled to the New World. Once here, the Europeans fused their medical knowledge with that of the Native Americans. Herbal know-how became an important part of early American habits, so that wellness remedies were handed down from mothers to daughters to granddaughters, and medicinal plants were grown in home gardens. Physicians from the 1600s, 1700s, 1800s, and early 1900s commonly used plants, such as arnica, echinacea, and garlic to heal patients. Herbs were listed as medicine in official publications such as the *United States Pharmacopoeia* (the definitive American listing) and the *National Formulary* (the pharmacist's handbook). With the creation of synthetic medications in the 1930s, herbal medicine began to wane.

Fortunately, Europeans and Asians never gave up their herbal remedies. Instead, they used them to complement synthetic medications. Their successes—combined with the desire of many Americans for alternatives to the high price tags and unforgiving side effects of synthetic drugs—have kept the world moving forward on a healthier herbal path.

WHAT IS SAW PALMETTO?

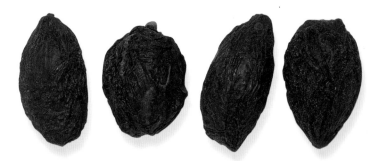

Though not as well known as certain herbal remedies, saw palmetto is rapidly gaining recognition for its ability to ease hormonal imbalances. Walk the aisles of any health food store and you can't miss it: saw palmetto in capsules, liquid extracts, teas, tinctures, and more. Yet saw palmetto is no medicinal newcomer—the herb boasts a long, distinguished history as a sexual aid, infection fighter, and diuretic. In fact, saw palmetto has been used by Native Americans for centuries to boost libido, enhance general wellness, and fight urinary tract infections.

European settlers to America became interested in the herb, and by the late 1800s and early 1900s, saw palmetto was a popular treatment for frequent urination and other symptoms associated with prostate enlargement and inflammation. Fortunately, when the American medical establishment abandoned saw palmetto in the 1950s for synthetic medications, physicians in France, Germany, and Italy continued to use the herb. Their success with it was great enough to influence their American counterparts and today, saw palmetto is an accepted treatment on both sides of the Atlantic for benign prostatic hyperplasia (BHP). In addition to the herb's antiandrogenic and antiestrogenic activities—which are directly responsible for treating BHP—saw palmetto also boasts anti-inflammatory actions. Furthermore, studies of small animal indicate that the herb also has antiallergenic and immune system-stimulating properties.

Saw palmetto is a small, hardy, palm tree native to the West Indies and the southeastern United States. It grows to 10 feet and is distinguished by long, swordlike leaf blades. The plant features deep red-brown to black, olive-sized fruit, called berries. These berries are wrinkled, oblong, with a diameter of 1/2 inch and a length of 1/2–1 inches. They are picked when ripe, then dried for medicinal use. Saw palmetto berries contain the plant's most important active components: saturated and unsaturated fatty acids and sterols.

IN OTHER WORDS
Like many herbs, saw palmetto is known by many names. Here are some of them:

* American Dwarf Palm
* Cabbage Palm
* Serenoa
* Serenoa repens

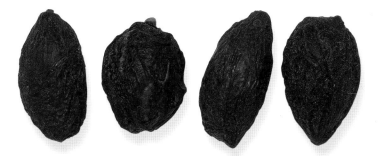

SCIENCE TALK

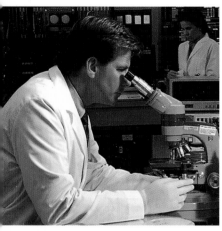

MEDICINE WORLDWIDE
The National Institutes of Health, in Bethesda, MD, estimate that only 10 to 30 percent of the health care worldwide is allopathic, or "Western." The rest of the world's medical care is what Americans would call "alternative," including ayurveda, energy healing, herbalism, homeopathy and traditional Chinese medicine.

CELEBRATING GERMAN KNOW-HOW
Perhaps no other country in the Western world has done more than Germany to further the cause of herbal medicine. What's the country's secret? Commission E, a review board of respected pharmacologists, physicians and scientists. The board was established in 1978, and members spent the first 15 years researching more than 300 age-old herbal remedies for usages, recommended dosages, preparations and side effects. Then, in 1980, the German government upped the medical ante, creating a mandate requiring all new herbal remedies sold in pharmacies to meet the same criteria as over-the-counter drugs. To comply, researchers performed thousands of rigorous clinical trials, resulting in a deep well of knowledge used by doctors open to herbs worldwide.

DO YOU HAVE A CONTRAINDICATION?

Before taking any herb, it's important to ask your physician whether you have any contraindications.

What does contraindication mean? It's a common medical term that refers to a symptom or condition that makes a particular treatment inadvisable. For example, because saw palmetto has documented hormonal actions, any hormone-dependent illness, such as estrogen-receptor-positive breast cancer, is a contraindication.

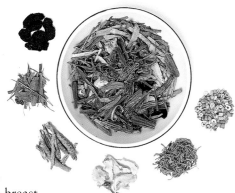

Before taking any herb, ask yourself the following questions:

✔ Have I done any background research on the herb?

✔ What condition am I taking this herb for?

✔ Am I taking other medications or herbs that may affect the herb's functioning?

✔ Do I have any pre existing condition that is contraindicated?

✔ Am I pregnant, trying to conceive, or nursing?

✔ Have I spoken to my physician, a naturopathic doctor or an herbalist before taking this herb?

✔ Do I know the proper dosages for the herb?

RETHINKING MEDICATION

ANTIBIOTICS: ARE THEY ESSENTIAL?

A recent report published in the *Journal of the American Medical Association* stated that even though antibiotics provide little help for colds, upper respiratory tract infections, and bronchitis, doctors still prescribe antibiotics for these conditions. Why? In part, because patients expect their doctors to give them some kind of medication, and many physicians find it easier to oblige than take time out to explain how antibiotics do and don't work. Americans are so enamored of antibiotics that doctors write over 12 million antibiotic prescriptions annually. To learn more about the dangers of antibiotic abuse, contact the Centers For Disease Control and Prevention, 404-332-4555.

PENICILLIN BY THE POUND

Since penicillin's debut in 1941, antibiotic production has shot up from 2 million pounds in 1954 to more than 50 million pounds in 1997. Where is all this medication going? Half of the antibiotics produced annually are prescribed for people; the rest are mixed into livestock feed and used as fertilizers for agricultural crops. The downside to this free-flowing penicillin? New, strong, antibiotic-resistant strains of bacteria.

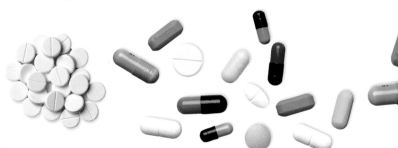

WAIT! BEFORE YOU TAKE THAT PILL . . .
Before asking your doctor for an antibiotic, ask yourself the
following questions:

✔ Is my condition caused by bacteria? If not, antibiotics
  will not work.

✔ Are antibiotics necessary for recovery? If the infection
  will go away on its own, consider forgoing antibiotics.

✔ Are there alternatives to antibiotics? If herbal or other
  natural remedies can fight off the infection, consider
  using one or more of them.

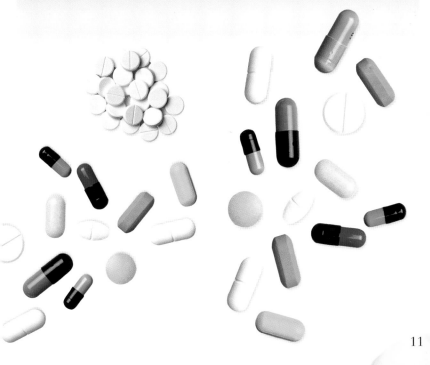

COMMON SIDE EFFECTS

Research shows that saw palmetto is remarkably safe, with no reported long-term toxicity. Infrequently, however, saw palmetto may cause mild side effects. Here's what a small number of users experience:

✔ Diarrhea. A very small number of individuals may experience diarrhea when using saw palmetto in dosages that are larger than recommended.

✔ Stomach Upset. A very small number of individuals may experience stomach upset when using saw palmetto in dosages that are larger than recommended.

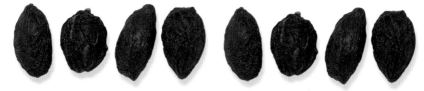

WHAT TO LOOK FOR
In the market for a saw palmetto remedy, but you're not sure how to choose one? Here's a hint: The most effective remedies boast a high concentration of active ingredients called fatty acids and sterols. To ensure that you get the most potent—and beneficial—medicine available, look for products standardized to 85 to 95 percent fat-soluble fatty acids and sterols per 160-mg dose.

PRECAUTIONS

✖ Saw palmetto should not be taken by individuals who are on prostate medicines.

✖ Do not take saw palmetto if you have a hormone-dependent illness such as estrogen-receptor-positive breast cancer.

✖ Saw palmetto should not be taken by individuals who are on hormonal treatments, including hormone replacement therapy and birth control pills.

✖ Saw palmetto should not be taken by women who are pregnant, trying to conceive, or nursing.

✖ To avoid dangerous interactions between prescription medication and herbal medicine, individuals with AIDS, cancer, a connective tissue disease, heart disease, kidney disease, liver disease, tuberculosis, or any other chronic illness should consult their physician before using any herb.

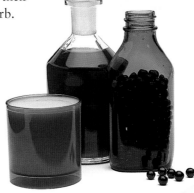

FORMULA GUIDE

Capsules, extracts, teas, tinctures—what do they all mean?
For the uninitiated, we offer this guide to herbal formulas:

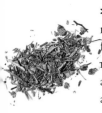

✻ Capsules. The medicinal part of the herb is freeze-dried, pulverized, and packed into gelatin capsules. Saw palmetto capsules usually contain 160 mg of herb powder; occasionally the dried herb is reinforced with concentrated extracts.

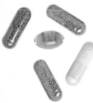

✻ Herb, Dried. The flowers, fruit, leaves, stems, and/or roots of many herbs are often available dried at health food stores and Chinese pharmacies. While these are most commonly made into homemade teas, they can also be used to make decoctions, infused oils, sachets, and more.

✻ Herb, Fresh. Herbs that are used in both culinary and medicinal ways (such as parsley or dill) are most often found fresh. These can be made into homemade extract, juice, infused oil, tea, and more.

✻ Juices. The extracted juice from fresh herbs can be found mixed with commercially prepared fruit or vegetable juices.

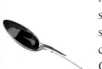

✻ Liquid Extract (also called Extract). Macerated plant material is steeped over a period of time in a solvent or solvents such as alcohol, glycerin, and/or water. The steeped liquid is then reduced to lessen the concentration of (or entirely remove) the solvents. Generally stronger than a tincture.

* **Oil, Essential** (also called Oil). Essential oils are the volatile oily components of herbs. They are found in tiny glands located in the flowers, leaves, roots, and/or bark and are mechanically or chemically extracted. Essential oil is prescribed almost exclusively for external use.

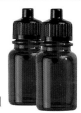

* **Oil, Infused.** Made by steeping fresh or dried herbs in an edible oil. After a period of time, the herbs are removed and the oil used internally or externally. Not as potent as essential oil.

* **Ointments.** Dried or fresh herbs are steeped in a base of oils and emulsifiers (such as beeswax, petroleum jelly, or soft paraffin wax). After a period of time, the herbs are removed and the ointment packaged. For external use only.

* **Syrups.** Syrups are usually a combination of herbal extracts and a sweetener, such as honey or sugar. Generally used for colds, flu, and sore throats.

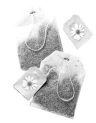

* **Teas/Infusions.** The words "tea" and "infusion" are often used interchangeably in herbal healing. While commercial herbal tea bags are available, herbal tea can also be made with loose dried or fresh herbs.

* **Tinctures.** Plant material is soaked in alcohol. The saturated plant material is then pressed. Liquid from this pressing may be diluted with water and packaged—usually in small dropper bottles.

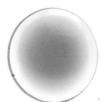

CONDITIONS AND DOSES

BENIGN PROSTATIC HYPERPLASIA

❒ **Symptoms:** The prostate is a walnut-sized gland responsible for contributing fluids to the semen. This protective fluid helps improve the survival of ejaculated sperm as it enters the vagina's acidic environment. As men age, however, it is common for the prostate gland to enlarge. In fact, according to a report by the National Institutes of Health, more than four of every five men between the ages of 50 and 60 suffer from an enlarged prostate. Called benign prostatic hyperplasia, or BPH in medical-speak, it is believed to be caused by an accumulation of testosterone in the prostate. Once within the prostate, testosterone is converted to the more potent hormone dihydrotestosterone (DHT).

DHT stimulates prostate cells to multiply, eventually causing the gland to enlarge. Why does this enlargement cause trouble? Not only does the prostate sit just below the bladder, it physically surrounds the urethra, the duct through which urine passes. Thus, when the prostate enlarges, it not only presses on the bladder, but also squeezes the urethra, creating symptoms such as decreased strength and force of urine stream, difficulty in initiating urination, dribbling after the end of urination, inability to sleep through the night without waking up to urinate, and frequent need to urinate.

❒ **How Saw Palmetto Can Help:** Saw palmetto's most documented usage—both historically and in modern medicine—is as a treatment for BPH symptoms. Anecdotal evidence from centuries of Native American and herbalist usage, plus hundreds of studies performed in the United States, Europe, and Japan, have shown that the herb strengthens urine flow, decreases the number of times needed to urinate, reduces residual urine, and makes it easier to initiate urination. Indeed, the herb has been shown in tests to exert anti-inflammatory effects. But the herb's main action in treating BPH is its ability to inhibit the conversion of testosterone to DHT.

❏ **Dosages:** If you experience any of the above symptoms, do not take saw palmetto without first visiting a physician for a medical diagnosis. Saw palmetto should not be taken by individuals who are currently taking medication for BPH. With a physician's go-ahead, take one 160-mg capsule of saw palmetto two times daily; or 1/2 teaspoon of liquid extract two times daily; or 1 teaspoon of tincture two times daily. In addition, you may drink up to 2 cups of saw palmetto tea daily. You should see mild improvement in four weeks, with more dramatic results after three months. Saw palmetto therapy can be continued as needed.

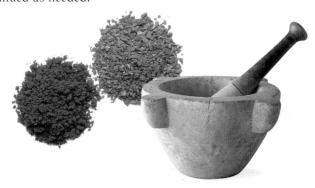

CONDITIONS AND DOSES

SAW PALMETTO TAKES ON THE COMPETITION

Individuals suffering from benign prostatic hyperplasia, or BPH, are often prescribed synthetic medication for their condition. However, more and more physicians—even physicians who would never think of recommending herbs—are going the natural route and prescribing saw palmetto. Why? Numerous studies pitting saw palmetto against synthetic medications have shown that saw palmetto is more effective—helping a greater percentage of patients, showing stronger results, and working in shorter amounts of time.

Proscar (finisteride) is currently the only approved synthetic drug to treat BPH. Like saw palmetto, it works by inhibiting the transformation of testosterone to dihydrotestosterone. Dihydrotestosterone—a very potent hormone derived from testosterone—is responsible for the overproduction of prostate cells, which ultimately results in prostatic enlargement. Yet fewer than 50 percent of patients on Proscar will experience clinical improvement after taking the drug for one year. Furthermore, it must be taken for at least six months before any improvement occurs.

Saw palmetto, on the other hand, has been shown in studies to benefit nearly 90 percent of patients, usually within four to six weeks. An example of just how effective saw palmetto is: After pooling data from 12 clinical studies, researchers found that after three months, patients on saw palmetto experienced a 38-percent increase in urine flow-rate per millisecond; those taking Proscar had to wait an entire year to reach a 16-percent improvement in urine flow-rate per millisecond.

ANOTHER USE

Androgen is a hormone found in both men and women, yet it's called a "male hormone" because it is found in much greater quantities in males. While small amounts of androgen are necessary for normal sexual development, too much can cause conditions such as hirsutism (excessive hair growth) or polycystic ovarian disease in women. Enter saw palmetto. The herb blocks androgen receptors in the body, thus inhibiting the formation of excess androgen. It is this antiandrogenic action that has led many experts to speculate about saw palmetto's ability to successfully treat androgen-excess conditions in women. Unfortunately, no formal studies have yet been completed. Stay tuned.

CONDITIONS AND DOSES

CYSTITIS

❏ **Symptoms:** Cystitis is an inflammation of the bladder. Commonly called a bladder infection, the condition is most often caused by *Escherichia coli*, a bacterium that lives in the intestines. Symptoms include cloudy urine that may contain blood, frequent urination, lower abdominal pain, an urgent desire to empty the bladder, and painful burning during urination.

❏ **How Saw Palmetto Can Help:** Saw palmetto has long been used by Native Americans to treat bladder infections. Indeed, the herb's fatty acids and sterols have been shown in clinical studies to reduce inflammation of the genitourinary tract and promote a more forceful flow of urine. In addition, the herb is believed to reduce the irritating quality of overly acidic urine, which is often associated with bladder infections. Studies of small animals also indicate that the herb stimulates the immune system, thus rousing the body's defenses against infectious organisms.

❏ **Dosages:** At the first sign of infection, take a 160-mg capsule of saw palmetto two times daily; or 1/2 teaspoon of liquid extract two times daily; or 1 teaspoon of tincture two times daily. In addition, you may also drink up to 2 cups of saw palmetto tea daily.

LOSE THE WATER
For centuries saw palmetto was used as an effective "water pill," prescribed by early American physicians, herbalists, and Native American healers. The herb exhibits strong diuretic qualities, helping the body to release trapped liquid through the urinary tract.

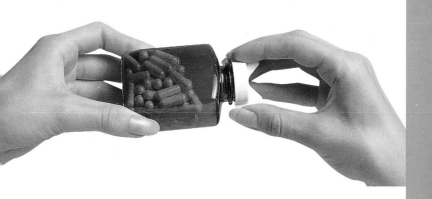

CONDITIONS AND DOSES

DYSMENORRHEA

❑ **Symptoms:** Mild to moderate pain during menstruation is normal and occurs when the uterus contracts to shed its temporary lining. However, sometimes the uterus contracts more than necessary, causing extreme pain. This condition is called dysmenorrhea. It is believed to be caused by excessive levels of prostaglandins. The primary symptom is strong to severe pain in the lower abdomen during menstruation; this pain may radiate to the hips, buttocks, or thighs. Other signs include diarrhea, dizziness, excessive perspiration, fatigue, nausea, and vomiting.

❑ **How Saw Palmetto Can Help:** Before the creation of synthetic drugs, saw palmetto was a popular menstrual aid. Saw palmetto is a tonic herb, which is said to both strengthen and relax the uterine muscles. Stronger and more relaxed uterine muscles translate to diminished uterine muscle contractions, and thus less pain. **Note:** Painful periods are not always a sign of dysmenorrhea. In some cases they signal an underlying disease, such as endometriosis. If you suffer from painful periods, please see your physician to rule out any existing illness.

❑ **Dosages:** At the first sign of symptoms, enjoy 1 or 2 cups of saw palmetto tea. For stronger relief, take one 160-mg capsule of saw palmetto two times daily; or 1/2 teaspoon of liquid extract two times daily; or 1 teaspoon of tincture two times daily.

THE FERTILITY FRUIT?
Infertility is defined as the inability to conceive after a
full year of unprotected intercourse. The problem can lie
with the male (up to 40 percent of all cases) or female
(up to 60 percent of all cases). Although medical
measures—fertility drugs, in vitro fertilization, donor
eggs or sperm—can increase the chance of conceiving,
medical intervention is costly, physically invasive, and
time-consuming. The alternative? Many herbalists claim
that saw palmetto has helped patients become pregnant
in the presence of unexplained infertility. Indeed, the herb
has historically been used to restore ovarian action and
strengthen testicle function. But does this mean saw
palmetto can make an infertile person fertile?
Unfortunately, no large-scale study has been done on the
subject. Right now, the medical establishment views saw
palmetto's fertility ability as anecdotal.

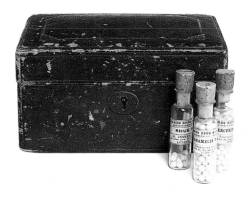

CONDITIONS AND DOSES

MENOPAUSE

❒ **Symptoms:** Menopause is not an illness but a natural condition that occurs when the ovaries no longer produce enough estrogen to stimulate the lining of the uterus and vagina sufficiently. Simply put, menopause is when women no longer menstruate or get pregnant. It generally occurs somewhere between the ages of 40 and 60. One of the most famous signs of menopause is the hot flash, a sudden reddening of the face accompanied by a feeling of intense warmth. Other common symptoms include depressed mood, fluid retention, insomnia, irritability, nervousness, night sweats, ovarian pain, painful intercourse, rapid heartbeat, susceptibility to bladder problems, tender uterus, thinning of vaginal tissues, vaginal dryness, and weight gain. It should be noted that some women experience few symptoms, while still others encounter none at all.

❒ **How Saw Palmetto Can Help:** One traditional "remedy" for menopause is hormone replacement therapy. This optional treatment uses synthetic hormones to elevate progesterone and estrogen to their premenopausal levels. Saw palmetto can be helpful regardless of whether one undergoes or forgoes hormone replacement therapy. According to saw palmetto's historic uses, the herb's fatty acids and sterols have a tonic effect on vaginal walls, ovaries, and uterine muscles. This helps prevent the vaginal tissue from thinning and becoming painfully dry, ovarian pains, and tender uterus that many menopausal women experience. Saw palmetto is also used to treat bladder infections, to which some menopausal women are prone.

❐ **Dosages:** Take one 160-mg capsule of saw palmetto two times daily; or 1/2 teaspoon of liquid extract two times daily; or 1 teaspoon of tincture two times daily. With your physician's recommendation, the same dosage can be taken as a complement to hormone replacement therapy.

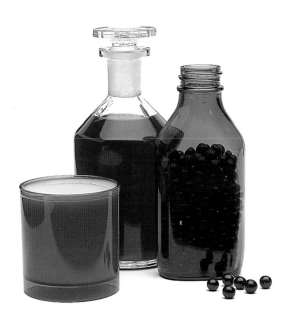

CONDITIONS AND DOSES

AN HERBAL BUST BOOSTER?

In Native American healing, saw palmetto was often prescribed to small-busted women who wanted to enlarge their breasts. Indeed, years of anecdotal evidence from early American doctors and herbalists have reported that with long-term usage—in this case, a year or more—mammary glands can sometimes grow slightly to moderately larger. Even modern studies have found that in very rare, isolated instances, men on saw palmetto experience a slight increase in breast size. It's important to note that saw palmetto doesn't have this effect on everyone, nor is it known exactly why the herb enlarges only some people's breasts. It is believed that saw palmetto hormonal actions, which in turn increase breast tissue. It is the herb's theorized hormonal activity that makes it off-limits for anyone with a hormone-dependent illness, such as estrogen-receptor-positive breast cancer.

BREASTFEEDING AID

These days, saw palmetto is most often associated with male sexuality—prostate conditions, in particular. But the herb has a long, documented history as a helper for more feminine conditions as well, including infertility, painful periods, menopause, and breastfeeding. In fact, both Native American healers and early American midwives prescribed saw palmetto to new mothers to start the free flow of breast milk, increase breast milk production, and protect lactating breasts from nursing hazards such as mastitis. Though modern studies have yet to be done on saw palmetto's affect on lactation, the herb continues to be used this way by many modern herbalists and midwives.

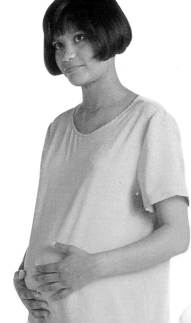

CONDITIONS AND DOSES

IMPOTENCE

❏ **Symptoms:** While anything from too much alcohol to anger or depression can cause short-term erectile problems, impotence is defined as a chronic inability in the presence of sexual desire to have or sustain an erection. It is believed that as many as 30 million American men suffer from the condition. In 90 percent of the cases, an organic cause is the culprit—usually diminished blood flow caused by fatty deposits in the arteries leading from the heart to the penis.

❏ **How Saw Palmetto Can Help:** In Native American medicine, saw palmetto was regularly used to treat impotence. In fact, it was historically prescribed to promote growth and nutrition to testicles that were "wasting" due to varicocele, a swelling of the scrotum caused by varicose veins. Although saw palmetto cannot help impotence caused by emotional issues, modern herbalists use the herb to tone and strengthen the male reproductive system. This, in turn, is believed to promote stronger erections.

❏ **Dosages:** Take one 160-mg capsule of saw palmetto two times daily; or 1/2 teaspoon of liquid extract two times daily; or 1 teaspoon of tincture two times daily. Continue therapy as needed.

A BERRY GOOD FOOD

Today saw palmetto is best known as a medicinal plant. Indeed, this is one of the ways Native Americans used this indigenous plant—as an aid for bladder infections, breastfeeding, impotence, infertility, and respiratory conditions. However, early Americans also ate ripe saw palmetto berries as fruit. The berries' flavor is alternately described as cloying, extremely sweet, or soapy.

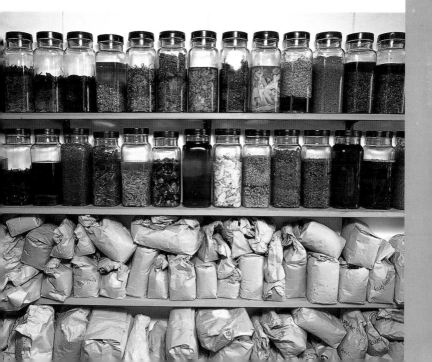

CONDITIONS AND DOSES

LOW LIBIDO

❏ **Symptoms:** Libido is a Latin word meaning "sexual drive." Today, if someone talks about a low libido (sometimes called frigidity), he or she is referring to a low desire for sex. Of course, there are many reasons one doesn't feel like having sex, including anger toward a partner, bad body image, fatigue, low self-esteem, negative attitude toward sex, physical illness, and more. Yet sometimes, there is no concrete reason.

❏ **How Saw Palmetto Can Help:** While saw palmetto has long been used by Native Americans and herbalists as an aphrodisiac, its effects are purely anecdotal; there have been no official studies examining the herb's effect on sexual desire. It is said that saw palmetto's tonic effects on the male and female reproductive system and the herb's hormonal actions both help produce a desire for sex. However, before trying saw palmetto, it's a good idea to examine any possible underlying causes for low libido— such as anger or low self-esteem.

❏ **Dosages:** If there is no reasonable explanation for low libido, take one 160 mg capsule of saw palmetto two times daily; or 1/2 teaspoon of liquid extract two times daily; or 1 teaspoon of tincture two times daily. Continue therapy as needed.

GETTING THE MOST MEDICINE

Saw palmetto's active ingredients are still a mystery to scientists. Whatever the compounds responsible for saw palmetto's medicinal actions, they seem to be located in the berries' fatty acids and sterols. When analyzed, these fatty acids and sterols were shown to contain capiric, caprylic, caproic, isomyristic, lauric, myristic, palmitic, oleic, and stearic acids; phytol, farnesol, geranylgeraniol, and polypheol alcohols; beta-sitosterol, carotenes, cycloartenol, ethyl esters, glucoside, lipase, lupeol, lupenonone, stigmasterol, 24-methylcycloartenol, and tannins. Scientists claim that because the majority of ingredients are fat-soluble, they do not dissolve in water; a fat-soluble substance such as alcohol or hexane is needed to extract them. Products that contain such substances include specially manufactured capsules made with fat-soluble saw palmetto extracts, liquid extracts, and tinctures.

All this may be so, agree many herbalists and Native American healers. But the plant also contains other unidentified beneficial ingredients which aren't fat-soluble—making decoctions, teas, and other home remedies effective. So which side has it right? Both undoubtedly have valid points. Thus, throughout the book, fat-soluble options are recommended, and instances where nonfat-soluble home remedies are appropriate are noted.

CONDITIONS AND DOSES

ACUTE BRONCHITIS

❏ **Symptoms:** Acute bronchitis is a common illness characterized by inflammation of the bronchi, the breathing tubes that lead to the lungs. Caused by the same virus responsible for the common cold, bronchitis is characterized by constriction of the chest, chest pain, coughing (often with yellowish sputum), difficulty breathing, fatigue, fever, and sore throat.

❏ **How Saw Palmetto Can Help:** One of saw palmetto's historic uses—by Native Americans, early American physicians, and country herbalists—was as a treatment for any type of coughing. In fact, many modern-day herbalists still use saw palmetto for coughing. The herb's fatty acids and sterols both soothe bronchial membranes and reduce inflammation of these membranes, alleviating discomfort and making breathing easier. Studies of small animals also indicate that the herb stimulates the immune system, thus rousing the body's defenses against infectious organisms.

❏ **Dosages:** At the very first sign of illness, immediately take a 160-mg capsule of saw palmetto two times daily; or 1/2 teaspoon of liquid extract two times daily; or 1 teaspoon of tincture two times daily. In addition, you may drink up to 2 cups of saw palmetto tea and take 3 tablespoons of saw palmetto syrup daily. Continue therapy until symptoms are gone.

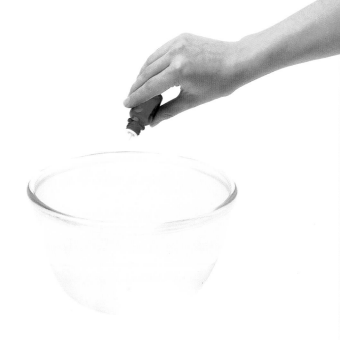

CONDITIONS AND DOSES

COLD

❐ **Symptoms:** Ever wonder why it's called the common cold? Because it is just that: common. In fact, it is estimated that healthy adults get an average of two colds per year. Most colds are caused by a rhinovirus, although in some instances bacteria can be to blame. Symptoms include coughing, nasal congestion, malaise, sneezing, sore throat, and watery eyes.

❐ **How Saw Palmetto Can Help:** Native Americans, early medical doctors, and country herbalists have historically used saw palmetto as a treatment for any type of coughing. Modern herbalists still use the herb for coughs. That's because saw palmetto's fatty acids and sterols both soothe and reduce inflammation of the bronchial and nasal membranes. The result? Less congestion and easier breathing. Studies of small animals also indicate that the herb stimulates the immune system, thus rousing the body's defenses against infectious organisms.

❏ **Dosages:** At the very first sign of illness, immediately take a 160-mg capsule of saw palmetto two times daily; or 1/2 teaspoon of liquid extract two times daily; or 1 teaspoon of tincture two times daily. In addition, you may drink up to 2 cups of saw palmetto tea and take 3 tablespoons of saw palmetto syrup daily.

To ease the sore throat that often accompanies a cold, gargle with saw palmetto tea or decoction up to three times daily. Continue therapy until symptoms are gone.

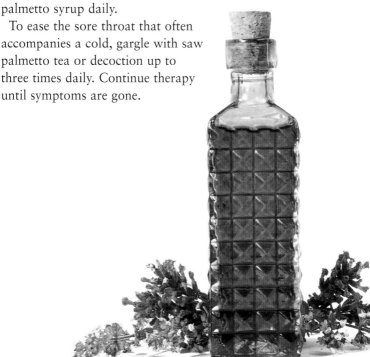

GATHERING YOUR OWN

Hunting wild herbs is a satisfying introduction to herbal therapy—but when done thoughtlessly, it can cause plant extinction. In fact, today's increased interest in wild herb gathering has left many indigenous plants extinct; echinacea, ginger, ginseng, goldenseal, sweet grass, and wild carrot are now nearly impossible to find in their native habitats. Fortunately, saw palmetto is safe for now—but to keep it that way, please ask yourself the following questions before gathering:

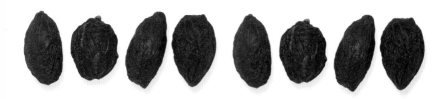

✔ Is this plant endangered? If so, it may be illegal in your state to gather it.

✔ Do I need to take this herb from the wild or can I purchase it or grow it myself?

✔ Am I gathering for personal use only and not for commercial use? **Note:** Gathering wild plants for commercial use is illegal in many states.

✔ What part of the plant do I need? Saw palmetto's berries contain the most concentrated percentage of active ingredients and are best gathered after warm weather has passed—September through January is when most saw palmetto berries are gathered. Aim for mid- to late-morning after the dew has dried.

✔ Do I know the plant's mode of reproduction? When gathering a plant that reproduces from seeds, random flowers or fruit must be left on each plant in order to generate more seed. When gathering an herb that reproduces from underground rhizomes, plants should be thinned evenly, leaving no discernible "bald patches."

✔ What will I be using this herb for and exactly how much of it do I need?

✔ Is the ground wet where the plant is growing? If so, find herbs growing in a dry spot or return when the ground is dry. Walking on wet soil compresses the dirt, making it difficult for future growth.

✔ Are the plants growing in sprayed areas, such as farmland sprayed with pesticides or marshes sprayed for mosquito control?

✔ Can I leave behind enough healthy plants for the local animal population?

✔ Can I leave behind enough healthy plants that can reproduce?

ALTERNATIVE HEALTH STRATEGIES

Herbs, vitamins, minerals—sure these contribute to good health. But creating general well-being involves more than simply taking supplements. Good health has to do with various quality of life issues that can aggravate or cause stress, thus harming health. Here are some additional ways to help keep yourself well.

Improve Your Eating Habits

Here are the five main eating strategies people follow; consider finding the healthiest one that works with your lifestyle.

- OMNIVORE
- PISCATORIAL
- MACROBIOTIC
- VEGAN
- VEGETARIAN

Get More Exercise

Whether it's walking or weightlifting, any type of exercise can help you feel better. Try any of these types:

- STRETCHING
- AEROBICS
- STRENGTH TRAINING

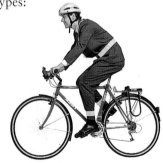

Simple Ways To Ease Stress

In addition to exercise and healthy eating, here are some more techniques–old and new–for easing stress and increasing relaxation.

- GET ENOUGH SLEEP
- MEDITATE REGULARLY
- GIVE UP JUNK FOOD
- ADOPT A PET
- SURROUND YOURSELF WITH SUPPORTIVE PEOPLE
- LIMIT YOUR EXPOSURE TO CHEMICALS
- TAKE YOUR VITAMINS
- ENJOY YOURSELF

ONE-MINUTE STRESS REDUCER

Stress is one of the top health hazards we face today. Unfortunately, it's impossible to go through life without the irritations that make us tense. Fortunately, there *is* something you can do to minimize their power to aggravate you. It's called deep breathing, and it can be done anywhere and anytime you need to calm and center yourself. Here's how it works:

1. Inhale deeply through your nose.
2. Hold your breath for up to three seconds, then exhale your breath through your mouth.
3. Continue as needed.

Deep breathing pulls a person's attention away from a given stressor and refocuses it on his or her breath. This type of breathing is not only comforting (thanks to its rhythmic quality), but also has been shown to lower rapid pulse and shallow respiration—two temporary symptoms of stress.

GET MOVING

Ask medical experts to name one stay-young strategy and there's a good chance "exercise" will be the answer. And with good reason. Exercise, whether a gentle walk around the block or a full-tilt weight lifting session, strengthens the heart, lowers the body's resting heart rate, builds muscles, boosts circulation to the body and the brain, revs up the metabolism and burns calories. All of which can keep a person look and feel his or her best. To be effective, exercise must be performed several times a week. Aim for at least three sessions. However, there's more than one kind of exercise. For optimum health, try a combination of aerobic exercise and strength training. And don't forget to stretch before and after each workout!

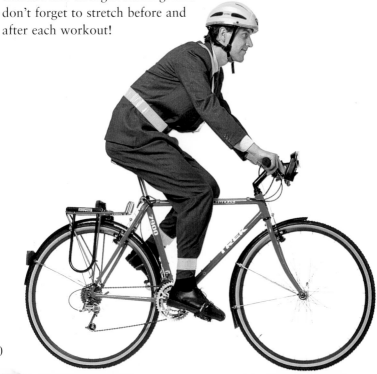

STRETCHING

❏ **What It Is:** Any movement that stretches muscles. Examples include bending at the waist and touching the toes, sitting with legs outstretched in front of you, and rolling your neck. Stretch for eight to twelve minutes before every workout and again after you exercise.

❏ **Why It's Important:** Muscles act like springs. If a muscle is short and tight, it loses the ability to absorb shock. The less shock a muscle can absorb, the more strain there is on the joints. Thus, stretching maintains flexibility, which in turn prevents injuries. Because we often lose our regular range of motion with age, stretching is especially important for older adults to prevent sprains, strains and falls.

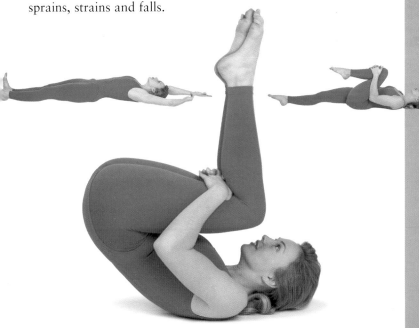

GET MOVING

AEROBICS

❑ **What It Is:** Any activity that uses large muscle groups, is maintained continuously for 15 minutes or more and is rhythmic in nature. Examples include aerobic dance, jogging, skating and walking. Ideally, you should aim for three to six aerobic workouts per week.

❑ **Why It's Important:** Aerobic exercise trains the heart, lungs and cardiovascular system to process and deliver oxygen more quickly and efficiently to every part of the body. As the heart muscle becomes stronger and more efficient, a larger amount of blood can be pumped with each stroke. Fewer strokes are then required to rapidly transport oxygen to all parts of the body.

STRENGTH TRAINING

❒ **What It Is:** Any activity that improves the condition of your muscles by making repeated movements against a force. Examples include lifting large or small weights, sit-ups, stair-stepping, and isometrics.

❒ **Why It's Important:** Strength training makes it easier to move heavy loads, whether they require carrying, pushing, pulling or lifting, as well as to participate in sports that require strength. The exercises are of various kinds. Some require changing the length of the muscle while maintaining the level of tension, others involve using special equipment to vary the tension in the muscles, and some entail contracting a muscle while maintaining its length.

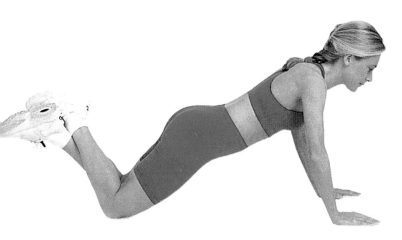

EATING SMART

A balanced diet is the foundation of good health. For proof, just read the numerous medical studies that link healthy eating with disease prevention and disease reversal. These same studies connect high fat intake, high sodium consumption and diets with too much protein to numerous illnesses, including cancer, cardiovascular diseases, diverticular diseases, hypertension and heart disease. But what exactly is a balanced diet? Generally speaking, it is a diet comprised of carbohydrates, dietary fiber, fat, protein, water, 13 vitamins and 20 minerals. More specifically, it is a diet built around a wide variety of fruits, legumes, whole grains and vegetables. Alcohol, animal protein, high-fat foods, high-sodium foods, highly-sugared foods, sodas and processed foods are consumed sparingly, if at all.

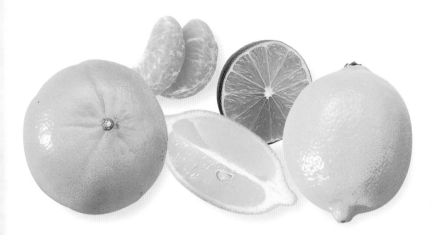

OMNIVOROUS

❏ **On The Menu:** Plant-based foods, dairy products, eggs, fish, seafood, red meats, organ meats, poultry.

❏ **Foods That Are Avoided:** None. Everything is fair game.

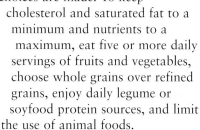

❏ **How Healthy Is It?** It depends. Someone who eats eggs, poultry or meat every day, chooses refined snacks over whole foods and gets only one or two daily servings of fruits and vegetables will not be as healthy as an omnivore who limits meat (the general dietary term for any "flesh foods," including poultry and fish) to two or three times a week, chooses water over soft drinks, and gets the recommended five or more daily servings of fruits and vegetables. Complaints about traditional omnivorous diets revolve around the diet's high level of cholesterol and saturated fat (found in animal-based foods), which increases one's risk of cancer, diabetes, heart disease and obesity. However, an omnivorous diet can be a healthy one, provided thoughtful choices are made. To keep cholesterol and saturated fat to a minimum and nutrients to a maximum, eat five or more daily servings of fruits and vegetables, choose whole grains over refined grains, enjoy daily legume or soyfood protein sources, and limit the use of animal foods.

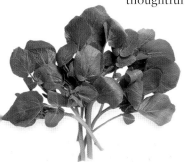

EATING SMART

PISCATORIAL

❏ **On The Menu:** Plant-based foods, dairy products, eggs, fish, seafood.

❏ **Foods That Are Avoided:** Red meats, organ meats, poultry.

❏ **How Healthy Is It?** Like an omnivorous diet, a piscatorial diet is as healthy as a person makes it. Individuals who eat high-fat and highly processed foods fail to get the recommended daily number of vegetables and fruits, and eschew whole grains for processed grains will not enjoy optimum health. That said, individuals who are conscientious about eating a balanced, varied diet, and who limit fish and seafood intake to two or three times per week, can expect a lower risk of heart disease, oily fish, especially since many oily fish contain omega-3 fatty acids. Eaten in moderation, has been found to help lower blood cholesterol. Be aware, however, that oily saltwater fish, such as shark, swordfish and tuna, have been found to carry mercury in their tissues; many health authorities recommend eating these varieties no more than once or twice a week. Also, due to overfishing, many fish species are now threatened, including bluefin tuna, Pacific perch, Chilean sea bass, Chinook salmon, and swordfish. For additional information on endangered fish, visit the University of Michigan's Endangered Species Update at www.umich.edu/~esuupdate, or the Fish and Wildlife Information Exchange at http://fwie.fe.vt.edu.

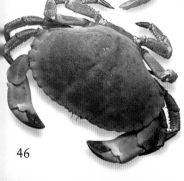

MACROBIOTIC

❏ **On The Menu:** Plant-based foods, fish, very limited amounts of salt.

❏ **Foods That Are Avoided:** Dairy products, eggs, foods with artificial ingredients, hot spices, mass-produced foods, organ meats, peppers, potatoes, poultry, red meats, shellfish, warm drinks, refined foods.

❏ **How Healthy Is It?** Macrobiotics is based on a system created inn the early 1900s by Japanese philosopher George Ohsawa. The diet consists of 50 percent whole grains, 20 to 30 percent vegetables, and 5 to 10 percent beans, sea vegetables and soy foods. The remainder of the diet is composed of white-meat fish, fruits and nuts. The diet's low amounts of saturated fat, absence of processed foods, and emphasis on high-fiber foods, such as whole grains and vegetables, may promote cardiovascular health. Because soy and sea vegetables contain cancer-fighting compounds, macrobiotics is often recommended to help treat cancer. However, critics worry that the diet's limited variety of food can leave followers lacking in certain vitamins and important cancer-fighting phytonutrients.

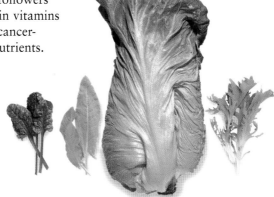

EATING SMART

VEGAN

❒ **On The Menu:** Plant-based foods.

❒ **Foods That Are Avoided:** Dairy, eggs, fish, seafood, red meats, organ meats, poultry. Also avoided are foods made by animals or processed with animal parts, such as gelatin, honey, marshmallows made with animal gelatin, white sugar processed with bone char.

❒ **How Healthy Is It?** A vegan (pronounced VEE-gun) diet can be extremely healthy. Like the vegetarian diet, a vegan diet has been shown by numerous studies to lower blood pressure and prevent heart disease. In addition, the high fiber intake cuts one's risk of diverticular disease and colon cancer. Yet, because vegans do not eat dairy products or eggs, they must be more conscientious than vegetarians about either eating plant foods with vitamin B_{12} and vitamin D, or taking supplements of these nutrients.

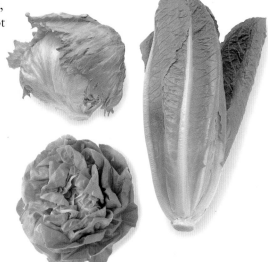

VEGETARIAN

❐ **On The Menu:** Plant-based foods, dairy, eggs.

❐ **Foods That Are Avoided:** Fish, gelatin, seafood, red meats, organ meats, poultry.

❐ **How Healthy Is It?** A vegetarian diet can be very healthy when done right. Fortunately, this isn't hard. Dietary science has debunked theories of "protein combining" popular in the 1960s and 1970s, leaving today's vegetarians to worry only about eating a wide variety of whole foods, including beans, fruits, grains, low-fat dairy products, nuts, soy foods, and vegetables. A varied daily diet insures enough protein, calcium and other nutrients for vegetarians of all ages, including children, pregnant individuals and the elderly. A well-chosen vegetarian eating plan has been shown by numerous studies to lower blood pressure, decrease one's risk of breast cancer and prevent heart disease. In addition, the diet's high fiber levels cuts the risk of diverticular disease and colon cancer.

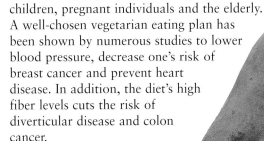

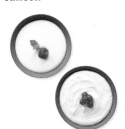

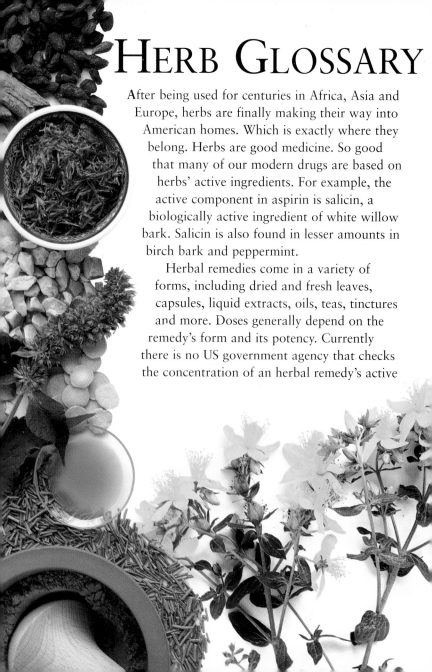

HERB GLOSSARY

After being used for centuries in Africa, Asia and Europe, herbs are finally making their way into American homes. Which is exactly where they belong. Herbs are good medicine. So good that many of our modern drugs are based on herbs' active ingredients. For example, the active component in aspirin is salicin, a biologically active ingredient of white willow bark. Salicin is also found in lesser amounts in birch bark and peppermint.

Herbal remedies come in a variety of forms, including dried and fresh leaves, capsules, liquid extracts, oils, teas, tinctures and more. Doses generally depend on the remedy's form and its potency. Currently there is no US government agency that checks the concentration of an herbal remedy's active

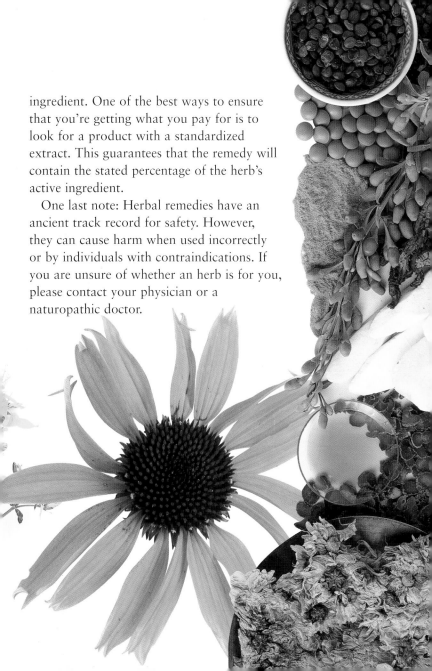

ingredient. One of the best ways to ensure that you're getting what you pay for is to look for a product with a standardized extract. This guarantees that the remedy will contain the stated percentage of the herb's active ingredient.

One last note: Herbal remedies have an ancient track record for safety. However, they can cause harm when used incorrectly or by individuals with contraindications. If you are unsure of whether an herb is for you, please contact your physician or a naturopathic doctor.

ALOE

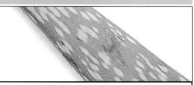

Properties: Analgesic, antibacterial, antifungal, anti-inflammatory, anti-itch, antiseptic, circulatory stimulant, digestive aid, immune-system stimulant, laxative.
Target Ailments: Acne, bruises, burns, constipation, cuts, insect bites, digestive disorders, rashes, ulcers, wounds.
Available Forms: Capsule, fresh leaves, gel, juice, liquid extract.
Possible Side Effects: When taken internally, aloe can cause severe cramping in some individuals.
Precautions: Pregnant women should not ingest aloe; It can stimulate uterine contractions.

CALENDULA

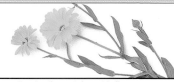

Properties: Antibacterial, anti-inflammatory, antiseptic, antispasmodic, promotes sweating, sedative.
Target Ailments: Burns, cuts, fungal infections, gallbladder conditions, hepatitis, indigestion, irregular menstruation, insect bites, menstrual cramps, mouth sores, skin rashes, ulcers, wounds.
Available Forms: Capsule, dried herb, fresh herb, liquid extract, lotion, oil, ointment, tincture.
Possible Side Effects: None expected.
Precautions: Calendula is related to ragweed. Individuals allergic to ragweed should consult a physician before using calendula.

ASTRAGALUS

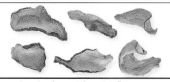

Properties: Antibacterial, anti-inflammatory, antioxidant, antiviral, diuretic, immune-system stimulant.
Target Ailments: Cancer, colds, appetite loss, diarrhea, fatigue, flu, heart conditions, HIV, viral infections.
Available Forms: Capsule, dried herb, fresh herb, liquid extract, tea, tincture.
Possible Side Effects: None expected.
Precautions: Astragalus should be used as a companion therapy to—not a replacement for—traditional cancer and HIV therapies.

CHAMOMILE

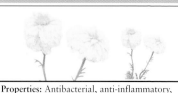

Properties: Antibacterial, anti-inflammatory, antiseptic, antispasmodic, carminative, digestive aid, fever reducer, sedative.
Target Ailments: Gingivitis, hemorrhoids, insomnia, indigestion, intestinal gas, menstrual cramps, nausea, nervousness, stomachaches, sunburns, tension, ulcers, varicose veins.
Available Forms: Capsule, dried herb, fresh herb, liquid extract, lotion, oil, tea, tincture.
Possible Side Effects: None expected.
Precautions: Because chamomile is related to ragweed, individuals with ragweed allergies should consult a physician before using chamomile.

DONG QUAI

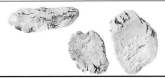

Properties: Antiallergenic, antispasmodic, diuretic, mild laxative, muscle relaxant, vasodilator.

Target Ailments: Abscesses, blurred vision, heart palpitations, irregular menstruation, light-headedness, menstrual pain, pallor, poor circulation.

Available Forms: Capsule, dried herb, liquid extract, tincture.

Possible Side Effects: Can cause photosensitivity in some individuals.

Precautions: Dong quai has abortive abilities; Do not take while pregnant.

FEVERFEW

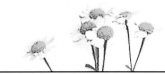

Properties: Anti-inflammatory, fever reducer.

Target Ailments: Arthritis, asthma, dermatitis, menstrual pain, migraines.

Available Forms: Capsule, dried herb, fresh herb, liquid extract, tincture.

Possible Side Effects: Some individuals experience "withdrawal" symptoms after taking feverfew, including fatigue and nervousness.

Precautions: Because it is related to ragweed, individuals with ragweed allergies should consult a physician before using feverfew.

ECHINACEA

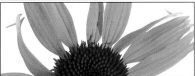

Properties: Antiallergenic, antibacterial, antiseptic, antimicrobial, antiviral, carminative, lymphatic tonic.

Target Ailments: Abscesses, acne, bladder infections, blood poisoning, burns, colds, eczema, food poisoning, flu, insect bites, kidney infections, mononucleosis, respiratory infections, sore throats.

Available Forms: Capsule, dried herb, liquid extract, tea, tincture.

Possible Side Effects: High doses can cause dizziness and nausea.

Precautions: Do not take echinacea for more than four weeks in a row.

GARLIC

Properties: Antibacterial, anticoagulant, antifungal, anti-inflammatory, antiviral, cholesterol reducer, digestive aid, immune-system stimulant, worm-fighting.

Target Ailments: Arteriosclerosis, arthritis, bladder infections, colds, digestive upset, flu, heart conditions, high blood pressure, high blood cholesterol, viral infections.

Available Forms: Capsule, fresh cloves, liquid extract, oil, tincture.

Possible Side Effects: Can cause upset stomach.

Precautions: While garlic is safe taken in culinary doses, individuals on anticoagulant medications should consult their doctors before supplementing their diet with garlic.

GINGER

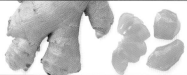

Properties: Antibacterial, anticoagulant, antinausea, antispasmodic, antiviral, carminative, digestive aid, expectorant, immune-system stimulant, muscle relaxant.

Target Ailments: Burns, colds, flu, high blood pressure, high cholesterol, liver conditions, intestinal gas, menstrual cramps, motion sickness, nausea, stomachaches.

Available Forms: Capsule, dried root, tea.

Possible Side Effects: Heartburn.

Precautions: While ginger is safe in culinary doses, individuals who suffer from a blood-clotting disorder or are on anticoagulant medication should consult a physician before supplementing their diet with the herb.

GINSENG

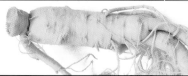

Properties: Antibacterial, antidepressant, immune-system stimulant, stimulant.

Target Ailments: Colds, depression, fatigue, flu, impaired immune system, respiratory conditions, stress.

Available Forms: Capsule, dried root, fresh root, liquid extract, tincture, tea.

Possible Side Effects: Large doses of ginseng can cause breast soreness, headaches or skin rashes in some individuals.

Precautions: Ginseng can aggravate existing heart palpitations or high blood pressure.

GINKGO BILOBA

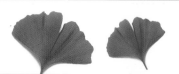

Properties: Antibacterial, anti-inflammatory, antioxidant, circulatory stimulant, vasodilator.

Target Ailments: Clotting disorders, dementia, depression, headaches, hearing loss, Raynaud's syndrome, tinnitus, vascular diseases, vertigo.

Available Forms: Capsule, dry herb, liquid extract, tincture, tea.

Possible Side Effects: Diarrhea, irritability, nausea, restlessness.

Precautions: Do not use ginkgo biloba if you have a blood-clotting disorder like hemophilia or are taking anticoagulant medications.

GOLDENSEAL

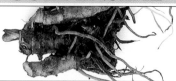

Properties: Antacid, antibacterial, antifungal, anti-inflammatory, antiseptic, astringent, digestive aid, stimulant.

Target Ailments: Canker sores, contact dermatitis, diarrhea, eczema, food poisoning.

Available Forms: Capsule, dry herb, liquid extract, tea, tincture.

Possible Side Effects: In high doses, goldenseal can cause diarrhea and nausea and can irritate the skin, mouth and throat.

Precautions: Because of its high cost, many manufacturers adulterate preparations with less costly herbs, such as barberry, yellow dock or bloodroot, some of which can cause unwanted reactions when taken in high doses.

KAVA

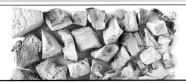

Properties: Antidepressant, antispasmodic, aphrodisiac, diuretic, muscle relaxant, sedative.
Target Ailments: Anxiety, colds, depression, menstrual conditions, muscle cramps, respiratory tract conditions, stress.
Available Forms: Capsule, dried herb, liquid extract, tea, tincture.
Possible Side Effects: Allergic skin reactions, muscle weakness, red eyes, sleepiness.
Precautions: In high doses, kava can impair motor reflexes and cause breathing problems.

MILK THISTLE

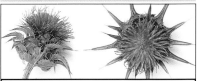

Properties: Anti-inflammatory, antioxidant, digestive aid, immune-system stimulant.
Target Ailments: inflammation of the gallbladder duct, hepatitis, liver conditions, poisoning from ingestion of the death cup mushroom, psoriasis.
Available Forms: Capsule, dried herb, fresh herb, powder, tea, tincture.
Possible Side Effects: Milk thistle can cause mild diarrhea when taken in large doses.
Precautions: If you think you have a liver disorder, seek medical advice before taking this herb.

LAVENDER

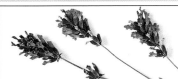

Properties: Antibacterial, antidepressant, antiseptic, antispasmodic, carminative, circulatory stimulant, digestive aid, diuretic, sedative.
Target Ailments: Anxiety, depression, headache, insomnia, intestinal gas, nausea, tension.
Available Forms: Capsule, dried herb, fresh herb, oil, tincture.
Possible Side Effects: Lavender products can cause skin irritation in sensitive individuals.
Precautions: Lavender oil is poisonous when ingested internally.

PARSLEY

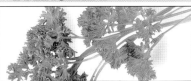

Properties: Antiseptic, antispasmodic, digestive aid, diuretic, laxative, muscle relaxant.
Target Ailments: Colds, congestion, fever, flu, indigestion, irregular menstruation, premenstrual syndrome, stimulating the production of breast milk, stomachaches.
Available Forms: Capsule, dried herb, fresh herb, liquid extract, oil, tea, tincture.
Possible Side Effects: Can cause photosensitivity in some individuals.
Precautions: Parsley should not be ingested in large amounts or used externally during pregnancy; it contains compounds that may stimulate uterine muscles and possibly cause miscarriage.

PEPPERMINT

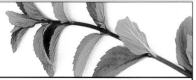

Properties: Antacid, antibacterial, antidepressant, antispasmodic, carminatve, expectorant, muscle relaxant, promotes sweating.
Target Ailments: Anxiety, colds, fever, flu, insomnia, intestinal gas, itching, migraines, morning sickness, motion sickness, nausea.
Available Forms: Capsule, dried herb, fresh herb, lozenge, oil, ointment, tea, tincture.
Possible Side Effects: When applied externally, peppermint products can cause skin reactions in sensitive individuals.
Precautions: If you have a hiatal hernia, talk to your doctor before using peppermint products externally or internally; the oil in the plant can exacerbate symptoms.

SAGE

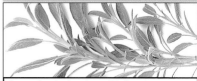

Properties: Antiseptic, anti-inflammatory, antioxidant, antispasmodic, astringent, bile stimulant, carminative, reduces perspiration.
Target Ailments: Excess intestinal gas, insect bites, menopausal night sweats, poor circulation, reduces milk flow at weaning, sore throat, stomachaches, mouth ulcers.
Available Forms: Capsule, dried herb, fresh herb, liquid extract, oil, tincture.
Possible Side Effects: Sage tea may cause inflammation of the lips and/or tongue in some individuals.
Precautions: Do not ingest pure sage oil; it is toxic when taken internally.

ROSEMARY

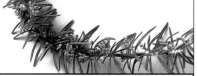

Properties: Antibacterial, antidepressant, anti-inflammatory, antiseptic, carminative, circultory stimulant.
Target Ailments: Bad breath, dandruff, depression, eczema, headaches, indigestion, joint inflammation, mouth and throat infections, muscle pain, psoriasis, rheumatoid arthritis.
Available Forms: Dried herb, fresh herb, ingestible rosemary-flavored oil, oil, ointment, tea, tincture.
Possible Side Effects: Rosemary oil can cause skin inflammation and/or dermatitis.
Precautions: Do not mistake regular rosemary oil for ingestible rosemary-flavored oil.

SAW PALMETTO

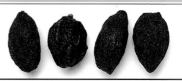

Properties: Antiallergenic, anti-inflammatory, diuretic, immune-boosting.
Target Ailments: Asthma, benign prostatic hyperplasia, bronchitis, colds, cystitis, impotence, male infertility, nasal congestion, sinus conditions, sore throats.
Available Forms: Capsule, dried herb, fresh herb, liquid extract, oil, tea, tincture.
Possible Side Effects: Can cause diarrhea if taken in large doses.
Precautions: Due to its hormonal actions, saw palmetto may interact negatively with prostate medicines or hormonal treatments such as estrogen replacement therapy, possibly canceling out their effectiveness.

ST. JOHN'S WORT

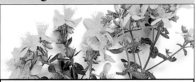

Properties: Analgesic, antibacterial, anti-depressant, anti-inflammatory, antiviral, astringent.
Target Ailments: Attention deficit disorder, anxiety, bacterial infections, burns, carpal tunnel syndrome, depression, HIV, menopause.
Available Forms: Capsule, dried herb, liquid extract, oil, ointment, tea, tincture.
Possible Side Effects: Gastrointestinal upset, headaches, photosensitivity, stiff neck.
Precautions: Avoid foods containing the amino acid tyramine when taking St. John's wort; the interaction of the two can cause an increase in blood pressure. Foods with tyramine include beer, coffee, wine, chocolate and fava beans.

WILD YAM

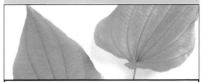

Properties: Analgesic, anti-inflammatory, antispasmodic, expectorant, muscle relaxant, promotes sweating.
Target Ailments: Menopause, menstrual cramps, morning sickness, nausea, rheumatoid arthritis, urinary tract infections.
Available Forms: Capsule, cream, dried root, liquid extract, oil, powder, tincture.
Possible Side Effects: Can cause vomiting in large doses.
Precautions: Individuals who are suffering from a hormone-sensitive cancer, such as breast or uterine cancer, should avoid wild yam. Some experts believe that the herb can encourage the growth of cancer cells.

VALERIAN

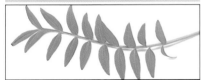

Properties: Analgesic, antibacterial, antispasmodic, carminative, reduces blood pressure, sedative, tranquilizer.
Target Ailments: Brachial spasm, high blood pressure, insomnia, palpitations, menstrual pain, migraines, muscle cramps, nervousness, tension headaches, wounds.
Available Forms: Capsules, dried herb, liquid extract, oil, teas, tincture.
Possible Side Effects: Headaches with prolonged use.
Precautions: Do not take with other sedatives, including alcohol. Do not drive or operate machinery after taking valerian.

YARROW

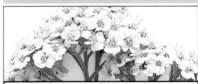

Properties: Antibacterial, anti-inflammatory, antispasmodic, blood coagulator, bile stimulating, immune-system stimulant, promotes sweating, sedative.
Target Ailments: Anxiety, colds and flu, cystitis, digestive disorders, menstrual cramps, minor wounds, nosebleeds, poor circulation, skin rashes.
Available Forms: Dried herb, capsule, liquid extract, oil, tea, tincture.
Possible Side Effects: Diarrhea, skin rash.
Precautions: Yarrow is related to ragweed and can cause an allergic reaction in individuals with ragweed allergies. Do not take if pregnant; it can induce miscarriage.

HERBAL TERMS

You're thumbing through the latest herbal therapy book when you run smack into the word "emmenagogue." Or perhaps you get tangled on "oxytocic." For anyone who's ever been stopped by an unfamiliar alternative medical term, we offer the following list:

Adaptogenic: Increases resistance and resilience to stress. Supports adrenal gland functioning.

Alterative: Blood purifier that improves the condition of the blood, improves digestion, and increases the appetite. Used to treat conditions arising from or causing toxicity.

Analgesic: Herb that relieves pain either by relaxing muscles or reducing pain signals to the brain.

Anthelmintic: Destroys or expels intestinal worms.

Antacid: Neutralizes excess stomach and intestinal acids.

Antiallergenic: Inactivates allergenic substances in the body.

Antibacterial/Antibiotic: Helps the body fight off harmful bacteria.

Antidepressant: Helps maintain emotional stability.

Anticatarrhal: Eliminates or counteracts the formation of mucus.

Anticoagulant: Thins blood and helps prevent blood clots.

Antifungal: Kills infection-causing fungi.

Anti-inflammatory: Reduces swelling of the tissues.

Anti-itch: Deadens itching sensations.

Antimicrobial: Kills a wide range of harmful bacteria, fungi, and viruses.

Antioxidant: Fights harmful oxidation.

Antipyretic/Fever Reducer: Reduces or prevents fever.

Antiseptic: External application prevents bacterial growth on skin.

Antispasmodic: Prevents or relaxes muscle tension.

Antiviral: Helps the body fight invading viruses.

Astringent: Has a constricting or binding effect. Commonly used to treat hemorrhages, secretions and diarrhea.

Blood Coagulant: Thickens blood and aids in clotting.

Carminative: Relieves gas.

Cholagogue: Encourages the flow of bile into the small intestine.

Circulatory Stimulant: Promotes even and efficient blood circulation.

Demulcent: Soothing substance, usually mucilage, taken internally to protect injured or inflamed tissues.

Diaphoretic: Induces sweating.

Diuretic: Increases urine flow.

Emetic: Induces vomiting.

Emmenagogue: Promotes menstruation.

Emollient: Softens, soothes and protects skin.

Expectorant: Assists in expelling mucus from the lungs and throat.

Galactogogue: Increases the secretion of breast milk.

Hemostatic: Stops hemorrhaging and encourages blood coagulation.

Hepatic: Tones and strengthens the liver.

Hypotensive: Lowers abnormally elevated blood pressure.

Immune-System Stimulant: Strengthens immune system so the body can fight off invading organisms.

Laxative: Promotes bowel movements.

Lithotriptic: Helps dissolve urinary and biliary stones.

Muscle Relaxant: Loosens tight muscles and reduces muscle cramping.

Nervine: Calms tension.

Oxytocic: Stimulates uterine contractions.

Rubefacient: Increases blood flow at the surface of the skin.

Sedative: Quiets the nervous system.

Sialagogue/Digestive Aid: Promotes the flow of saliva.

Stimulant: Increases the body's energy.

Tonic: Promotes the functions of body systems.

Vasoconstrictor: Constricts blood vessels, limiting the amount of blood flowing to a particular area.

Vasodilator: Dilates blood vessels, helping to promote blood flow.

Vulnerary: Encourages wound healing by promoting cell growth and repair.

HERBAL ORGANIZATIONS

Where to go for more information:

American Botanical Council
P.O. Box 201660
Austin, TX 78720
512-331-8868
www.herbalgram.org

The American Herbalist Guild
P.O. Box 746555
Arvada, CO 80006
303-423-8800

American Herbalists Guild
Box 1683
Soquel, CA 95073
408-464-2441

Herb Research Foundation
1007 Pearl Street, Suite 200
Boulder, CO 80302
303-449-2265
www.herbs.org

National Accupuncture and Oriental Medicine Alliance
14637 Starr Road SE
Olalla, WA 98359
206-851-6896

National Institutes of Health Office of Alternative Medicine
9000 Rockville Pike
Building 31, Room 5B-37
Mailstop 2182
Bethesda, MD 20892
301-402-2466

The Herb Society of America
9019 Kirtland-Chardon Road
Kirtland, OH 44094
216-256-0514

American College of Sports Medicine
P.O. Box 1440
Indianapolis, IN 46206
317-637-9200

National Health Information Center
P.O. Box 1133
Washington, DC 20013
800-336-4797

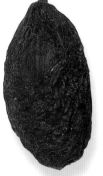
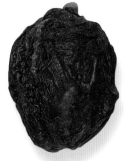

GROWING HERBS

Interested in cultivating herbs yourself?
These sources can supply roots, plants, and/or seeds.

Catoctin Mountain Botanicals
P.O. Box 454
Jefferson, MD 21755
301-473-4351

Companion Plants
7247 N. Coolville Ridge Rd.
Athens, OH 45701
614-593-3092
E-mail: complants@frognet.net

Dry Fork Herb Gardens
R.R.#1 Box 21
Rockport, IL
217-437-5281

Ecofriendly Farms
15488 Barn Rock Rd.
Mendota, VA 24270
540-466-8689

Goodwin Creek Gardens
P.O. Box 83
Williams, OR 97544
541-846-7357

Herbal Exchange
P.O. Box 429
9160 Lentz Rd.
Frazeysburg, OH 43822
614-828-9968

Horizon Herbs
P.O. Box 69
Williams, OR 97544
541-846-6233
www.chatlink.com/~herbseed
E-mail: herbseed@chatlink.com

Johnny's Seeds
Rt. 1 Box 2580
Foss Hill Rd.
Albion, ME 04910
207-437-9294
www.johnnyseeds.com

Mountain Traditions
H.C. 68, Box 193
Big Creek, KY 40914
606-598-6904

Nature's Cathedral
Rt. 1 Box 120
Blairstown, IA 52209
319-454-6959

Prairie Moon Nursery
Rt. 3, Box 163
Winona, MN 55987
507-452-1362

Wilcox Natural Products
P.O. Box 391
755 George Wilson Rd.
Boone, NC 28607
828-264-3615
www.goldenseal.com

Wild Wonderful Farm, Inc.
P.O. Box 256
Franklin, WV 26268
212-736-1467

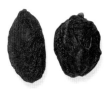

INDEX

ABOUT THE AUTHOR

Stephanie Pedersen is a writer and editor who specializes in the area of health. Her articles have appeared in numerous publications, including *American Woman, Sassy, Teen, Weight Watchers* and *Woman's World.* She has also co-written *What Your Cat is Trying to Tell You: A Head-to-Tail Guide to Your Cat's Symptoms and Their Solutions* and *What Your Dog is Trying to Tell You: A Head-to-Tail Guide to Your Dog's Symptoms and Their Solutions,* both published by St. Martin's Press. She currently resides in New York City.

Picture Credits: Steve Gorton, David Murray, Dave King, Martin Norris, Philip Gatward, Andy Crawford, Philip Dowell, Clive Streeter, Peter Chadwick, Tim Ridley, Andrew Whittack, Martin Cameron
Cover image by Steve Foster 1999

DORLING KINDERSLEY, INC.
www.dk.com

Published in the United States by
Dorling Kindersley, Inc.
95 Madison Avenue • New York, New York 10016

Copyright © 2000 by Dorling Kindersley, Inc.

Editorial Director: LaVonne Carlson
Project Editor: Nancy Burke
Designer: Carol Wells
Cover Designer: Gus Yoo

Pedersen, Stephanie.
    Saw Palmetto : hormone enhancer / by Stephanie Pedersen. --
    1st American ed.
    p. cm. -- (Natural care library)
    ISBN 0-7894-5335-5 (pbk. : alk. paper)
    1. Saw palmetto--Therapeutic use.   I. Title. II. Series.
RM666.S28P43 2000
615'. 3245--dc21
99-43069